VALERIE SMITH

Water, Fitness & Rehabilitation

The Easiest Way To Get Fit, Rehabilitate, Build Strength, and Improve Mobility, Strength and Flexibility. Low Impact Alternatives to Traditional Workouts

Exercise does not have to equal pain but water movement equals relief!

Valerie Smith

Contents

1

Introduction

I n our collective quest for a healthier, more vibrant life, we often overlook the simplest solutions nature offers us. Water, with its gentle resistance and buoyancy, provides a unique environment for exercise that is both effective and nurturing. It offers a unique blend of fitness, strength training, and therapeutic benefits, making it an ideal choice for individuals at any stage of their fitness journey. This book is your invitation to explore the transformative world of pool exercises, a realm where the goal of achieving improved mobility, flexibility, and overall well-being is not only attainable but also enjoyable.

I am someone who has always believed in the power of movement as medicine. Inspired by my own journey, my passion for helping adults of all ages achieve a healthier lifestyle through low-impact water workouts has only deepened over the years. My dedication to making fitness accessible and enjoyable for everyone, regardless of their skill level or physical condition, is the cornerstone of this book.

"Water Fitness and Rehabilitation" is crafted to be your companion, guiding you through the world of aquatic fitness with ease and clarity. It's designed with you in mind, offering a practical, inclusive, and supportive resource that resonates with anyone looking to begin or enhance their fitness journey. This book explores the benefits aquatic fitness can provide individuals at different levels of age, fitness, and health conditions. What sets this book apart is not just its comprehensive coverage of pool exercises but its dedication to ensuring that these workouts are accessible and enjoyable for all. Whether you are suffering from arthritis, diabetes, recovering from an injury, or just looking to improve your overall health, aquatic exercises are the most low impact alternative to traditional workouts. They aim to improve fitness, gain/regain strength and flexibility, manage pain, and enhance mobility without stressing your joints.

As we "dive" into the content, you'll gain an understanding how basic pool exercises can enhance your health and aid recovery. I will be interchanging "aquatics" and "hydrotherapy" throughout the book and both mean the use of water for exercise and/or rehabilitation. From improving flexibility and building strength to enhancing mobility, the impact is real and attainable. More than just teaching you about pool exercises, this book aims to motivate and inspire. It seeks to empower you with the knowledge and confidence needed to take control of your health and to stick with your aquatic fitness journey. The goal is not only to encourage you to start but also to support you every step of the way, ensuring that pool exercises become a cherished part of your lifestyle.

As we set forth on this journey together, I invite you to approach this book with an open mind and a readiness to embrace the transformative power of water workouts. Pool exercises are for everyone. Whether you have access to a simple community pool or a personal one, the possibilities for enhancing your health and wellness are limitless. No fancy equipment or previous experience is required—just a willingness to "dive" in (not literally).

I am genuinely excited about the journey that lies ahead for you. Approach this book with an open mind and a readiness to embrace the transformative power of water workouts. Rest assured, comprehensive guidance and support await you within these pages. Together, let's make waves in your fitness journey, one splash at a time.

2

The Magic Of Water

Before we begin diving into the aquatic exercise themselves, it is important for you to understand the benefits of buoyancy and its advantages for fitness and recovery. Buoyancy reduces the strain on joints and muscles, making exercises more accessible for individuals with mobility issues or injuries. Although buoyancy makes movements easier, water resistance ensures workouts remain challenging, promoting strength and endurance building. Many traditional exercises can be adapted to the pool, leveraging buoyancy for reduced impact and increased effectiveness. An added benefit is that the sensation of water can have calming effects, reducing stress and enhancing the overall exercise experience.

The key to hydrotherapy or aquatics is that water provides natural resistance in all directions, which can be adjusted by changing the speed and surface area of movements. By altering techniques and equipment, individuals can customize the intensity of their workout to fit their fitness levels and goals. The resistance encountered in water exercises engages multiple muscle groups simultaneously, offering a comprehensive workout. The resistance offered by water makes it an ideal medium for rehabilitation exercises, aiding in the recovery of injuries without additional strain.

3

Equipment

Whether or not you have your own pool or you choose to go to a community pool, aquatics is a simple way to provide optimum success with or without equipment. The best part of aquatics is there are many different workouts that do not require any equipment and the method of performing the exercises determines the level of intensity workout you will do. If you choose to use equipment, rest assured, most equipment is affordable to most. For instance, you can purchase a pool noodle at a local store for a range of $1-$3. You can order/purchase low cost equipment at a pool store or on Amazon. Pool noodles are a great and low cost equipment that helps you float while working your lower extremities. They also can be used to provide resistance to your upper arms. Kick boards help you float on your stomach and kick behind you and you can get two kick boards for $14.99. Aquatic dumbbells help for strength training and rehabilitation and can be purchased for as low as $19.99. In addition, there are many other options that can be tailored to your desire for level of fitness or your stage in your recovery process. Floatation devices, such as vest or back straps, a pool noodle, kick board or ankle cuffs, can help someone in deep water have proper form without worrying about having to wade the water. Remember, never jump in a pool wearing a floatation device or resistance equipment. Although the equipment is not necessary, incorporating equipment can intensify your water workouts, target specific muscle groups, and add a variety to your routines. Further chapters will incorporate equipment and show various options for all workouts with the hopes of encouraging creativity and fun in your workout routines. Remember, use of floatation devices should be determined by a person's strength, stability and swimming abilities. With proper supervision and knowing your own abilities, safety should be able to be obtained effortlessly.

Choosing the proper clothing for being in water is very important. Never wear any loose fitting clothing when doing exercises. This will weigh you down sometimes making it difficult to pull yourself up out of water. Fun fact, however, against what you would think, wearing long sleeve clothing designed for water exercises can help maintain the regulation of body temperature. If you do not have one of these, a bathing suit or tight tank tops or tight fitting biker shorts would be a good option. You can do aquatics with or without shoes, but always make sure if you do use shoes, they are water shoes, not regular sneakers. Water shoes will ensure the water flows not weighing down your legs. According to the AEA, shoes are recommended for those pregnant, obese, with diabetes or with musculoskeletal disorders (muscles, bones, tendons, ligaments, joints, and cartilage disorders). Shoes help provide traction and proper alignment during exercises. Aqua fitness equipment is meant to be safe if used properly. Always obtain physician approval prior to initiating exercise or when significantly altering an existing exercise program.

4

Water Temperature

We are now going to dive into equipment safety, starting with water temperature and depth safety. The Aquatic and Exercise Association (AEA) developed a Standards and Guidelines for Aquatic Fitness Programming and included information that there are certain water temperatures ideal for certain water exercise activities. The proper water temperature will help prevent injury. As we will see, warm ups will help maintain proper body temperature, but beginning with proper water temperature is a safe way to ensure you are not taxing your body unnecessarily. Please use this guide when determining whether your pool or community pool is right for your needs.

- **Arthritis**: 83-90 / 28.3-32.2 °C (91 - 94 F (32.8 - 24.4 C) may be allowed with special considerations*)
- **Children**: 83-86 / 28.3-30 °C
- **Children Swim Lessons**: 84+ / 28.9+ °C (Varies with age, class length, and programming; ideal to learn to swim programs are best suited for 84-89 / 28.9-31.7 °C when available)
- **Competitive Swimming**: 78-82 / 25.6-27.8 °C

- **Infant Programs (4 & under)**: 90-93 / 32.2-33.9 ℃
- **Multiple Sclerosis**: 80-84 / 26.7-28.9 ℃
- **Obese**: 80-86 / 26.5-30 ℃
- **Older Adults**: 83-86 / 28.3-30 ℃ (Moderate to High Intensity)
- **Older Adults**: 86-88 / 30-31.1 ℃ (Low Intensity)
- **Parkinson's Disease**: 90-92 / 32.2-33.3℃ (Ideal temperature)
- **Pregnancy**: 83-85 / 28.3-29.4 ℃ (Note: This range has been shown by research that indicates this range is safe for pregnancy, but the upper limit for safe water temperature has not been identified).
- **Resistance Training**: 83-86 / 28.3-30 ℃ (Minimum Range)
- **Therapy & Rehab**: 90-95 / 32.2-35 ℃ (Low function program – cooler temperatures may be more appropriate for higher intensity programs and specific populations)

Other important information in the AEA "Standards and Guidelines for Aquatic Fitness Programming" identifies the importance of water depth. Water Depth will determine the impact or weight bearing stress on the body. Each workout will identify the proper depth of water, but know that shallow water reduces the impact on the body while allowing for control of the body. These workouts can still work all body muscles and joints but know that water depth below waist level workouts will need to alter the intensity to avoid injury to joints and muscles. In addition, be forewarned that waist high water does not allow for the water to cool the body during exercise so intensity should be adjusted when doing exercises in shallow water. Depths of 3-5 feet is recommended and be careful when exercising near the slopes to deeper areas of the pool. Deep water exercises is ideal in water depths of 6.5 feet or more.

When checking heart rates during aquatic exercising, know that heart rate is lower while exercising in water so a great way to determine if you are working too hard is by monitoring your discomfort or fatigue during exercising.

Listening to music is a great way to pass time when exercising and music during pool exercises is no different. One thing to be cautious of though is that moving to the beat while in water can sometimes have you distracted that you will be working your body too hard. For most individuals, it is best to move your arms or legs to every half beat, rather than every beat. For those of you who are already at a high level of fitness, go for it and jam out to what keeps you moving.

Arms under water build muscle and help develop balance. Arms under water treading water helps both with stability and gives a great upper body workout. It is not recommended to raise your arms above water if you have spine or shoulder issues. You should not abruptly move arms in and out of water. Exercises should either be fully immersed or fully out of water, not the combination of the two. Hand held weights should be used intermittently and you should be taking a break between reps.

5

Tailoring Your Water Routine Based on Age and Ability

I cannot express more the importance of tailoring pool exercises to individual abilities, ages, and fitness levels for maximum benefit and safety. For instance, those recovering from a knee replacement will not be able to do the same intensity of exercises as someone who has been going to land gyms for months. Likewise, those stroke victims will not be able to do the intense levels of exercise as those who are recovering from a knee replacement. You must be sure to talk to your doctor, know your body and limitations, and identify if you need a partner in the water with you at all times. If you take all of these things into account, then you will have no problem completing any of the exercises within your category of need. It is important to not overdo your workouts at first and listen to your body. You should have rest periods and implement the recovery exercises in your pool routine. It is a good idea to use a progress tracker regardless of if you are doing this for rehabilitation purposes or to help with your overall health. As you progress further or as your goals change, you may begin to incorporate more advanced methods, or move onto other exercises you find interesting and entice you to keep going on your physical journey.

The workouts can be implemented by most everyone as long as you recognize the stage of your journey!

6

Managing Health Conditions

Arthritis and Joint Pain Relief

As you know, having arthritis is oftentimes debilitating. Doing everyday tasks may be impossible for you. If you have Osteoarthritis, then you most likely haven't been able to walk, run or do aerobic activities for years. Having conditions such as this impedes your ability to exercise. Your joints do not have the same cushioning that those without osteoarthritis have. Those with arthritis have chronic pain with movements and joints ache, unlike those who do not have arthritis. For this reason, aqua therapy is the best option for you to get exercise. Studies show that when you are in waist high water, you release pressure on your joints by 50% and when you are in neck high water, you release pressure on your joints by 90%. Water provides a series of gentle, fluid movements designed to enhance joint flexibility and reduce pain. Hydrostatic Pressure, or immersing your body in water, provides gentle pressure during exercises that can help reduce swelling and improve circulation. Sounds great, doesn't it? Journaling the benefits you feel will help motivate you to keep going so I encourage you to do that.

Sample Exercises for Joint Pain:

5-10 Minutes
  Warm up

Straddle yourself in the water with your shoulders just under the water. Bring your arms out to the side forming a "T", then **roll your head to the side**. Bring your arms down slowly, then raise them again to a T position. Roll your head to the other side. Repeat for 10 reps.

Then roll instead of rolling your head left to right, you will now **roll your head attempting to touch your ear with your shoulder**. Then next rep roll to the other side attempting to touch your ear with your shoulder. Do slow movements and do what feels good. Do not do it so you feel pain. Aquatic exercise is supposed to be painless, so don't be afraid that you are not pushing yourself enough. Results still come!

Next you will do a **forward arm reach**. You will be in a straddled position with your shoulders just under the water. You will reach forward as far as you can go, then reach back as far as you can go. Do this for 10 reps. Again, with time, your reach may or may not become further, but that is not the goal. You are working your body to lower your swelling and pain, so worrying about that progression is not important.

Workout

Next you will do a **diagonal arm reach**. In a straddle position with your shoulders just under the water, you will reach diagonal while lowering your body in a deeper straddle allowing your body to move in the direction of the reach. . Raise yourself back up to a starting position and reach to the other side, again lowering your body in a deeper straddle. Repeat for 10 reps.

Next you will do a **diagonal arm reach**, but out of the water. While in a straddle position with your shoulders just under the water, you will reach out of the water in a diagonal direction, then to the other side, then back into the water. Repeat for 10 reps.

Next you will do a **smooth stationary chest stroke** . Lower your body so your shoulders are just under the water, and begin to do a breast stroke. You will not be swimming, you will be stationary. Continue for 30 reps.

Next you will do cross arms. Lower your body so your shoulders are just under the water, and begin to cross your arms out in front of you. While having your arms maintain the same height, then bring them back behind you.

That was just a sample of what you can do but the exercises are endless. You can do wrist exercises if your arthritis in your wrists. Motions such as rolling your wrists, or doing an "opening a door knob" motion will help get you movement. Remember movement is medicine. Other examples are having your arms extended and then touching your fingers to your shoulders, or waving motions at your knuckles. Simply opening your hands and closing them while under water, or doing thumb circles. For your hips, you can float and move your legs side to side, or rotate at the hip and do leg lifts. You would be amazed how painless movements can be under water compared to out of water. I could go on and on with examples, but watching YouTube videos would give you numerous ideas!

Back Pain

Aquatics has an amazing ability to strengthen back muscles and improve spine health without the risk of injury. Just like joint pain, back pain can be a result of the spine compressing on nerves or other vertebrae in the back. So as with joint pain, with 50% of body weight being lifted off the joints in waist high water and 90% of weight being lifted off joints in neck high water, the same holds true for the back. Imagine being able to do relaxing exercises that do not cause pain, yet strengthens the back muscles and the core. Seems impossible, doesn't it? I know when you are suffering with back pain, it may appear so, but it is not impossible. By introducing core-focused exercises, you will be providing the necessary support and stability for a healthy back. And remember, I mentioned relaxing exercises, right? Well by doing relaxing and stretching exercises that leverage water's soothing properties helps to alleviate back pain too.

Heart Health and Improved Circulation

Everyone benefits from ways to improve heart health and circulation despite your level of physical health. Immersing your body in water increases central blood volume, decreases heart rate, increases cardiac output, and decreases diastolic blood pressure, which can last for hours. In addition, studies have shown that those with Congestive Heart Failure with associated Type II Diabetes have had benefits from aquatic exercise. Those with these conditions traditionally have poor oxygen output and weaker strength. After 8 weeks of training in water shoulder deep for 45 minutes 3 times a week, those patients were found to have better shoulder strength, stronger heel movements, and stronger work rate and walking abilities. Disclaimer, those with diabetes need to be careful with open wounds and in the one study, one patient wearing shoes developed a blister, which became problematic and that patient had to discontinue the program. However, those with neuropathy are advised to wear shoes. Always be sure to identify personal issues and consult with a doctor before beginning a program.

Managing Diabetes

Individuals with Type II Diabetes often have a weight factor. The Aquatic and Exercise Association suggests aqua fitness as a means to get stagnant individuals moving without excessive strain on the body and heart. Those who exercised for 12 weeks had found that their fasting glucose levels decreased (lowering the overall A1C levels by 1.1). They lowered their body weight, body fat, resting heart rate and blood pressure.

Rehabilitation and Recovery

As with any program involving injury, it is important to check with your doctor to ensure aquatic therapy is right for you. Rest assured though, studies show that the benefits of aquatic therapy are numerous for those in recovery stages from injuries or surgeries. Aquatic therapy is good for fractures, sprains, broken bones, joint surgeries, and ACL tears/repairs. It results in an ability to work on recovery earlier since water reduces body weight by 50-90% based on the depth of the pool. It results in a reduction of pain and swelling. It allows for the patient to work on proper gait, build strength and enhance cardiovascular health. Rehabilitation and recovery is definitely done in stages and the exercise in this book can be modified to more intensive workouts easily. Be sure to work with your physician or physical therapist to develop a program that is right for your level of injury or recovery.

Safety is always most important. Be sure to make sure you have others with you to help you get in and out of the pool and ensure proper technique when doing exercises. In the early stages of the recovery, be sure to do gentle controlled movements to avoid injury. You should feel confident, however, that aquatic therapy is one of the most pain free methods of rehabilitation. You must be patient, because with most surgeries, the recovery period can be anywhere from 4-20 weeks. Progressing slowly, and according to your doctor's recommendations will result in the best outcomes. Don't overdo it initially and gradually increase your intensity and duration in the pool to avoid overexertion and promote optimal healing.

Below is a sample of a program that can be incorporated for lower knee recovery or lower joint pain. Besides a warm up and cool down, these exercises do not need to be done in the same order. Also, there are many great sample videos on YouTube available for you to do your own research to help change up your programs. I highly recommend checking them out!

Example Lower Knee Recovery or Lower Joint Pain (Beginner):

5 min. warm up
  Walking in Waist High Water

Be sure to start with your feet firmly on the floor of the pool. Begin walking slowly by starting on your heels and rolling your weight to your toes. Push off with your toes. Keep your arms above water.

20 steps
  Walking in Waist High Water Incorporating Arms

Continue walking while incorporating your arms. With an open hand, put your arms down at your side and push both arms back at the same time while stepping. Keep your hands in the same position and pull your arms forward with the next step.

10-15 steps
Walking in Waist High Water With More Intensity

Continue walking with arms down in the water but with your hands cupped. Push both arms back at the same time while stepping. Turn your cupped hands towards the front of your body and pull your arms forward with the next step. You should feel more resistance with cupped hands.in Waist High Water

10 steps
Knee Raises in Waist or Mid Chest High Water

Walk forward being sure to start on your right heel and rolling your weight to your toes. Push off with your toes as you raise your left leg to a 90° angle. Slowly lower your left leg down, touching your heel first to the ground. Begin to roll your left foot from heel to toe while raising your right leg to a 90° angle and slowly lowering your right leg down touching your heel first to the ground.

10 reps
Knee Lifts to Leg Lift in Waist or Mid Chest High Water

Stand against the side of the pool. Raise your right leg to a 90° angle. Straighten your leg out slowly and gently lower it down by touching your heel to the ground. Raise the other leg to a 90° angle. Straighten your leg out slowly and gently lower it down by touching your heel down.

5-10 minute

Cool Down

Grab a pool noodle, a kick board or hold onto one of the steps. Adjust yourself to a floating position and kick your legs underwater for 5-10 min. Speed is not necessary. This is a cool down and this exercise should be relaxing.

Example Lower Knee Recovery or Lower Joint Pain (Intermediate):

5 min. warm up
  Walking in Waist High Water

Be sure to start with your feet firmly on the floor of the pool. Begin walking slowly by starting on your heels and rolling your weight to your toes. Push off with your toes. Keep your arms above water.

30 steps
  Walking in Waist High Water Incorporating Arms

Continue walking while incorporating your arms. With an open hand, put your arms down at your side and push both arms back at the same time while stepping. Keep your hands in the same position and pull your arms forward with the next step.

20 steps
  Walking in Waist High Water With More Intensity

Continue walking with arms down in the water but with your hands cupped. Push both arms back at the same time while stepping. Turn your cupped hands towards the front of your body and pull your arms forward with the next step. You should feel more resistance with cupped hands.

30 steps
Knee Raises in Waist or Mid Chest High Water

Walk forward being sure to start on your right heel and rolling your weight to your toes. Push off with your toes as you raise your left leg to a 90° angle. Slowly lower your left leg down, touching your heel first to the ground. Begin to roll your left foot from heel to toe while raising your right leg to a 90° angle and slowly lowering your right leg down touching your heel first to the ground.

20 steps
Side Steps in Waist or Mid Chest High Water

Stand with both feet on the floor of the pool shoulder width apart. Side step one leg at a time bringing yourself back to shoulder width apart. If you wish to get more of a challenge, squat down with each step. If you wish to include cardio, lower your arms into the water reaching to touch each hand on the opposite knee when stepping to the side and bringing the arms to water level when returning to shoulder width apart. Do not raise your arms high over your head when coming out of water if you have shoulder injuries.

15 steps
Lunges in Mid Chest High or Shoulder Deep Water

Stand in a lunging position being sure your front knee is not overextended over the front toes. Roll your front foot to your toes and push off rotating to lunge with your other leg and repeat.

20 steps
Gentle Jog in Mid Chest High or Shoulder Deep Water

Jog in place or by moving through the water alternating your arms with each step. If your goal is to add cardio, cup your hands while pulling the water back and forth.

5-10 minute
Cool Down

Grab a pool noodle, a kick board or hold onto one of the steps. Adjust yourself to a floating position and kick your legs underwater for 5-10 min. Speed is not necessary. This is a cool down and this exercise should be relaxing.

Example Lower Knee Recovery or Lower Joint Pain (Advanced):

5 min Warm up.
Walking in Waist High Water

Be sure to start with your feet firmly on the floor of the pool. Begin walking slowly by starting on your heels and rolling your weight to your toes. Push off with your toes. Keep your arms above water.

40 steps
Walking in Waist High Water Incorporating Arms

Continue walking while incorporating your arms. With an open hand, put your arms down at your side and push both arms back at the same time while stepping. Keep your hands in the same position and pull your arms forward with the next step.

20 steps
Walking in Waist High Water With More Intensity

Continue walking with arms down in the water but with your hands cupped. Push both arms back at the same time while stepping. Turn your cupped hands towards the front of your body and pull your arms forward with the next step. You should feel more resistance with cupped hands.

20 steps
Knee Raises in Waist or Mid Chest High Water

Walk forward being sure to start on your right heel and rolling your weight to your toes. Push off with your toes as you raise your left leg to a 90° angle. Slowly lower your left leg down, touching your heel first to the ground. Begin to roll your left foot from heel to toe while raising your right leg to a 90° angle and slowly lowering your right leg down touching your heel first to the ground.

30 steps
Side Steps in Waist or Mid Chest High Water

Stand with both feet on the floor of the pool shoulder width apart. Side step one leg at a time bringing yourself back to shoulder width apart. If you wish to get more of a challenge, squat down with each step. If you wish to include cardio, lower your arms into the water reaching to touch each hand on the opposite knee when stepping to the side and bringing the arms to water level when returning to shoulder width apart. Do not raise your arms high over your head when coming out of water if you have shoulder injuries.

15 steps
Lunges in Mid Chest High or Shoulder Deep Water

Stand in a lunging position being sure your front knee is not overextended over the front toes. Roll your front foot to your toes and push off rotating to lunge with your other leg and repeat.

20 steps
Walking Backwards in Waist or Chest High Water.

Walk backwards by touching your toe to the ground and roll to your heel. Alternate legs. Use your arms to balance. To increase intensity, increase your speed by being sure to be able to maintain balance at the same time.

40 steps
Gentle Jog in Mid Chest High or Shoulder Deep Water

Jog in place or by moving through the water alternating your arms with each step. If your goal is to add cardio, cup your hands while pulling the water back and forth.

5-10 minute
Cool Down

Grab a pool noodle, a kick board or hold onto one of the steps. Adjust yourself to a floating position and kick your legs underwater for 5-10 min. Speed is not necessary. This is a cool down and this exercise should be relaxing.

25

7

Interval Training for Strength and Toning

s with any exercise program, interval training gives better cardiovascular fitness. This can be incorporated into aquatic exercises in the same way as your land exercises. By alternating timing, intensity levels, and different parts of the body, you can achieve great results. Choosing high intensity exercises results in greater strength and fat burning. Although it is not necessary to incorporate weights into your program, it can help you get to your goal faster. Things such as hand fins, hand weights, pool noodles, etc, can add a form of further resistance in your hand movements, that result in better strength training. Simple tasks such as cupping your hands when you move your hands through the water, or moving faster in your motions can have some of the same results. As with any exercise program, the more you put into it, the more you get out of it. The great thing about aquatic exercise though is that you do not have to go through as much "pain and suffering" to achieve the same results as you would with land exercises. Tracking your progress can best help determine if timing or intensity has to be changed. Be sure to use a tracking program to help you stay on track and achieve your fitness goals. Feel free to use any of the combination of exercises below by doing 30 seconds on, 30 seconds off resting for 2 minutes between reps. It is recommended to start with 2 reps of the circuit and work your way up to 8 reps.

High Intensity Intermittent Workouts and Strength and Toning: Running

In waist high water, begin a running motion to each side of the pool being sure to touch your heels to the ground and rolling onto the balls of your feet. Pump your arms as you push through the water.

Increase Intensity:

Wear webbed gloves or cup your hands while pumping your arms; Hold a weighted object at chest level such as a weight or a kick board; use ankle weight for pools.

Leg Kicks

While holding onto the side of the pool and floating on your back, while keeping your leg as straight as possible, kick your legs up out of the water until your toes reach just out of the surface. Make sure your body is horizontal in the water by engaging your core.

Increase Intensity:

Use ankle weights approved for pools.

Squats

In waist high water, stand with legs shoulder width apart. Squat down in the water bringing your arms down to your side. Jump up lifting yourself out of the water while raising your arms to shoulder height. Go down to an immediate squat position again resisting your arms against the water back down to your sides as you go down.

Increase Intensity:

Hold pool weights in your arms. Do not bring your arms to shoulder height, just keep your arms down at your side.

Arm Flexes

Squat in waist high water. Use a kickboard and pull it into your chest with it in a vertical position. With force, push it out away from your chest and immediately back into your chest. Be sure to keep your core engaged.

Push ups

Stand facing the edge of the pool. Place your hands on the edge of the pool while placing your body in a plank position. Slowly lower your chest down and up mocking a push up on land.

Jumping Jacks

Stand with your legs should width apart in waist high water. Do a basic jumping jack by pushing and pulling your arms in and out of the water.

Increase Intensity:

Hold water weights in your arms while doing the jumping jack. Do not bring the weights down into the water, just to the top of the water.

Side Shuffles

Stand in shoulder height or waist high water. Shuffle from one side of the pool to the other. Be sure to keep your back straight and your core tightened.

Increase Intensity:

Wear pool approved ankle weights.

Leg Kicks

Stand facing the side of the pool with both feet on the bottom of the pool. Kick one leg back at a time alternating legs quickly.

Increase Intensity:

Wear pool approved ankle weights

Arm Curls

Squat down in the waist or shoulder high water. Use a pool noodle in the shape of a rainbow with both hands on each end at the top of the water. Pull the noodle down into the water until your elbows are into your belly.

Jump Rope

In waist high water, use a pool noodle and pull the noodle down into the water while bringing your knees to your chest to allow for the noodle to come around to your back. Pull the noodle out of the water from behind your head and continue that motion.

8

Mindfulness, Recovery and Nutrition

As with any fitness program, it is important to stay hydrated and consume enough calories for optimum recovery. Be sure to hydrate before, during and after exercising. If you are in the pool and you are getting foot or leg cramps, discontinue the exercise for that day. Make sure you hydrate more the next day before returning to the pool.

Set goals that are reasonable and achievable. Do not expect too much of yourself whether you are looking to get fit or you are working on recovering. Don't be too hard on yourself if you do not progress as fast as you thought. Keep a positive attitude and know you can do it! If you get bored, switch things up by trying different versions of the exercise. You can do combinations of upper body series, lower body series, knee exercises if your knees are sore that day. The possibilities are endless! As I said earlier, research videos on YouTube for other suggestions of exercises to keep it interesting for you. Getting a pool partner is a great idea to help keep you motivated and accountable. Stick to it and you will achieve much more success than if you do the work on land! Stay positive!

I am very happy to provide you with a quick reference book to aquatic exercises. If you like what this book has to offer, please leave a positive review and best of luck on your journey to greatness!

32

9

Resources

Resources

Aquatic Fitness Programming Standards and Guidelines. (n.d.). https://aeawave.org. Retrieved February 23, 2024, from https://aeawave.org/Portals/0/AEA_Cert_Docs/AEA_Standards_G uidlines_2020.pdf?ver=2019-12-18-131623-417%C3%97tamp=1576 696862726#:~:text=AEA%20recommends%20that%20deep%2Dwate r,specifically%20designed%20for%20water%20exercise

Cole, A., MD. (n.d.). *Water therapy for osteoarthritis.* Arthritis-health. https://www.arthritis-health.com/treatment/exercise/water-therapy -osteoarthritis

Dukovac, N. (2022, April 28). *10 pool exercises that help alleviate back pain.* Fairway Chiropractic Center. https://fairwaychiropractic.com/ blog/10-pool-exercises-alleviate-back-pain/

Feeback, S., ATRIC; Miriam Leary PhD, ACSM-CEP; Lori Sherlock EdD, ATRIC, CSCS.

(2019). *Aquatic Exercise for Individuals with Type 2 Diabetes Mellitus.* https://aeawave.org. Retrieved February 23, 2024, from https://aeawave.org/Portals/0/Research/Aquatic%20Exercise%20for%20Individuals%20with%20Type%202%20Diabetes%20Mellitus..pdf?ver=2019-06-17-161900-520×tamp=1560802911063#:~:text=In%20type%202%20diabetes%2C%20individuals,decreasing%20fasting%20blood%20glucose%20levels

Fetters, K. A. (2023, February 13). *7 pool exercises that burn fat fast.* EverydayHealth.com. https://www.everydayhealth.com/healthy-living/fitness/8-pool-exercises-burn-fat-fast/

Kim. (2023, September 25). *Water exercises to improve balance, Reduce fall risk - Master Spas blog.* Master Spas Blog. https://www.masterspas.com/blog/water-exercises-for-balance/

Lengacher, S. (2022, October 13). *Benefits of immersion on cardiac patients.* Hudson Aquatic. https://www.hudsonaquatic.com/benefits-of-immersion-on-cardiac-patients/

Poirier-Leroy, O. (2023, January 26). 6 best pieces of water exercise equipment for crushing your pool workouts - YourSwimLog.com. *YourSwimLog.com.* https://www.yourswimlog.com/best-water-exercise-equipment/

SneezeIT. (2021, January 5). *7 tips for overcoming a fear of swimming.* The Wave Aquatic & Fitness Center. https://www.whitefishwave.com/2021/01/7-tips-for-overcoming-a-fear-of-swimming/

Torres-Ronda, L., & Del Alcázar, X. S. I. (2014). The Properties of Water and their Applications for Training. *Journal of Human Kinetics, 44*(1),

237–248. https://doi.org/10.2478/hukin-2014-0129

Water Exercises for arthritis | Arthritis Foundation. (n.d.). https://www.arthritis.org/health-wellness/healthy-living/physical-activity/other-activities/hit-the-pool